My Sister's Story

Once was More than Enough

By Nicky Hawkins

Copyright Page

Table of Contents

My Sister Story "Once was More than Enough"

Foreword
By Johnny "Macknificent" Mack

I remember when we first started hearing about HIV and AIDS. I was newly married and living in California. It seemed like the crack epidemic was exploding and then we started hearing about AIDS. Initially the diagnosis was fatal and people were dying at enormous clips.

At first it was thought that it was a disease that affected homosexual men due to their risky behavior. It soon became evident that there were several different methods of transmission, one of which was a blood transfusion that the patient may not have been aware they have been exposed to the virus.

Another frightening and disheartening method of transmission was drug sharing needles.

People were frightened, they thought that if you touched an individual, if you kissed them, if you had any type of bodily fluid contact it would transmit the virus. Whole communities and cultures shifted their normal activity to make sure that they didn't spread or get infected with this deadly disease. Being careful has always been one attribute that I considered lifesaving.

Because my activities never hinged on that which would cause me to be exposed to the virus I felt like many that it was unnecessary for me to be aware of this scourge on humanity. Sure all over the years I watched the debate from green monkeys to government designed cultural decimation conspiracy theory. But deep down I felt as many that it was something that didn't affect me.

Affected people around me began succumb to the disease. I realized that it was larger than just a specific community like homosexuals or shared needle drug use that was being affected by this.

Whole families and communities were being destroyed because there was no cure or no control for what seemed to be the new plague of the 20th century. Around the world and even within the United States there was a state of caution. The end of that was the thought they could begin to at least control or limit the spread.

I have known Nicky Hawkins for at least 20 years. She has always been a quality, focused young lady that was always about her business. When I received the manuscript for Sonya's Story I was literally blown away. To know that someone that I knew was having to experience and deal with this debilitating disease at such a close range caused my heart to go out to her.

The Saga of Sonya's story is one that could be anyone's story. The fact that her sister Nicky Hawkins decided to leave a legacy that expressed her life is something that I find amazing. The drive, energy, and determination to make this a reality has caused people from many walks of life to give into making this dream become a reality.

I now have a profound sense of honor, respect, and admiration for Miss Nicky Hawkins for stepping out on faith and giving up her own home to make Sonya's House Inc a reality. But more importantly remember that Sonya was a real person who lived a real life and got caught up in a part of it that turned deadly.

The purpose of Nicky writing this book was to raise awareness about the AIDS virus and also to raise funds to make sure that those who are affected by it, in her care at least receive care, dignity, and a little peace before losing hope. Do your best and make sure that Sonya's House is able to continue doing it' best.

Johnny "Macknificent" Mack

Publisher

Dedication

This Book is dedicated to my Sister Sonya Kaye Thompson and the countless other sisters, mothers, aunts, cousins and friends who are dealing with AIDs

Why My Life Is Not My Own

Sonya's House founded in 2016, celebrates the life and spirit of Sonya Thompson. After 11 years of fighting, Sonya lost her battle from complications related to AIDS. Along her journey, she had difficulty accepting and compliance with her daunting medication regimen. From her experience while caring for Sonya, the founder recognized the need for support within the Dallas Community and has heeded its call. No one should endure this battle alone and we are here to help.

Opening 2017, this boarding house facility specializes in working with people affected by the virus that causes HIV and AIDS. We recognize the difficulty in adjusting to this life altering change; which can be mental, spiritual, physical and financial. Our goal is to provide low income housing and holistic care during this time.

Here at Sonya's House we want every individual affected by this illness to live life abundantly. In memory of Sonya, we will be there as partners on this journey. If you would like to learn more about Sonya's House please contact the Founder Nepfrintina Hawkins.

My Sister's Story

Once was more than enough!

My sister Sonya was an incredible, enlightened and giving big sister. She meant the world to me as she was to my older brother and to our mother. We all make choices in life and some of those choices can be destructive and oftentimes they are instructive. How do you begin to tell the story of someone's life that was senselessly cut so short?

No, I'm not talking about the destruction of the streets, or other random gun violence that is taking so many lives of our young people. I'm talking about something more sinister and a lot more preventable. In the next few pages I want to share the story of my sister and how one mistake not only cost her life, but also devastated the lives of everyone she knew and loved.

My name is Nicky Hawkins, I've worked in the medical field for over 20 years, and raised two incredible children Destiny and Christopher. My mother, Mary Thompson raised three kids of her own while working three jobs, consequently she was absent from the home most of the time. That left us to raise ourselves but not without the guidance and provision that mom so generously and lovingly provided.

My brother Joe, went to the penitentiary at age 21 for 12 1/2 years. He was released just four months before the passing of my sister Sonya. She has two kids, Erica and James and five grandkids. Of my siblings, Sonya was the oldest then Joe and myself.

We had a normal childhood as normal childhoods go. Mom provided a good upbringing. We came from good stock and we were absolutely delighted of that fact. We were very proud to be able to grow up in a loving, caring, decent household that provided the image of Christ and promoted education and morality.

Before Sonya's passing mom said that she didn't know how to be a mother. All she knew was to work and provide for us in the best way she could. She was committed to taking excellent care of us so we didn't lack or need anything. Sonya, my sister babysat Joe and me. My brother went to stay with his godparents at age 15 leaving Sonya and I to grow up with little to no adult supervision.

That led me to counseling three separate times for abandonment issues because there were no restraints, there was no significant guidance or processes in place for my sister and me. We just learned in love, which mom allowed us to. Although we did not have the normal restraints we still knew right from wrong and followed the structure that was in place, lax though it was.

As result of that unrestrained childhood I became a ultra-strict mother. All my life I've been very involved in my kid's life and they know it, share it and see it even today. On the other hand, I was allowed to do whatever I wanted because there was no one there to discipline my sister or me really. I skipped school and just enjoyed life as a child without any regards.

One of the cool caveats of that type of carefree life was all my friends could visit whenever they wanted and could spend the night without any questions. When mom came home and saw them there, her concern was to make sure enough food was in the house.

The truth is I wanted more discipline in my childhood because I thought discipline meant love. But all in all, I did not blame my mother for her lack of creating boundaries that children need to understand. Instead I love her even more because she gave me the independence and the power to be able to think for myself. Mom's greatest gift to us was **provision** not **pre-vision**, watching over or oversight. I can say that both my sister Sonya and I forgave her for not being there for us as kids.

The one unforeseen blessing of that limited infrastructure was confidence enough to engage in life without fear or some of the restraints that mentally held other kids in bondage.

We were always a close-knit family. Sonya had two kids and she was very involved in their education. She attended South Oak Cliff High School and upon graduation went to a community college. She taught school at a Learning Center Academy.

Sonya loved kids. She was the neighborhood mom. She taught for over 10 years. Although she was a single mom, all of her children had the same father. I share that as a significant back story.

My Sister Story "Once was More than Enough"

Looking for love

Far too many of us start looking for love in all the wrong places and all the wrong faces. He spent quality time with her kids and as I stated earlier, she was the neighborhood mom. I would just hang out at her house because of her attentiveness and quality lifestyle. It was a nurturing and fun environment. With all of that being said, she was also strict and respected. Everyone in the neighborhood came over to hang out.

In 1992 some 25 years ago, Sonya was living in an apartment and I would often go over there and visit. She was *saved*, super saved. She belonged to a holiness church and drove the school van. Her life consisted of no makeup and a very restricted holy lifestyle… long dresses with a dour expression and appearance. Sonya was the type of person that didn't just hang out as other kids or young people her age did once she gotten saved. Sonya was someone I admired and respected

Apartment life can be very unique and can cause too much conflict and confusion. One cause of conflict and confusion was a old man named Bobby who lived in the complex. **Bobby was a pimp.** In other words, he encouraged young girls to prostitute themselves for money and he would collect most if not all of it for himself. My cousin became one of his girls at the age of 15 begins prostituting herself in the service of Bobby.

Consequently, she got pregnant but miscarried. We all thought that Bobby was the most despicable person in the neighborhood.

He was always in and around Sonya's life and I often questioned her whether or not she slept with him. She gave me the same answer, ***"no, never not ever"***. That's the back story of what led to the inevitable result of what the book is about. My sister Sonya contracted AIDS and HIV.

My Sister Story "Once was More than Enough"

Denial Doesn't Make It Untrue

Sonya continually and adamantly denied having any type of sexual relationship with Bobby. One day she called to set us down to give us some depressing and disturbing news. The news was that she was HIV positive and it had been because of her sexual experience with Bobby. I was incredulous *how can Bobby give you AIDS when you never slept with him???*

Sonya then responded, *"Well I did"*. She was adamant about sharing this information with us as the virus was beginning to have an effect on her. She told us how she had got behind on her rent and went to Bobby for the rent money. In exchange for that rent money she slept with him, Just **Once**. Once was more than enough. Sonya had contracted HIV from him and now it was beginning to take its toll on her. It was rumored that Bobby went back to a small town in Louisiana where the disease finally got the best of him and he passed away.

My cousin also contracted the AIDS virus and she died tragically years later. But I'm getting ahead of myself. Sonya began going back-and-forth to the doctor and she would use my mother's car to do it. At first, we were not concerned but then it became so regular that we begin questioning her as to what was the nature of her illness? She initially told us that she had fibroids and had to undergo a procedure to remove them.

During this medical crisis, she was in position where she was not able to afford the rent any more. She moved out of that apartment and moved in with my mother. Isn't that ironic, fear of losing her apartment and then giving in to that sexual experience with Bobby and she still ended up losing the apartment

One day mom found a card on the front door from the health department indicating that Sonya needed to call them. Mom didn't want to confront her but I came over to mom's house and indicated that there had been a note on the door regarding her health. At that time she was in a relationship with someone else.

She finally came clean months later and sat us all down to tell us of her grim diagnosis.

She sat us down and shared the entire story. *"I got behind in rent and Bobby offered to pay it and bring me up* to date *if I slept with him. I agreed and we had a three-minute sexual encounter in which I didn't even have an orgasm but he did, isn't that ironic"* she said.

"Did Bobby pass away"? "Yes" then she said, *"he didn't get killed, he died of AIDS. He moved back to Louisiana when he got sick"* and he only weighed 96 pounds when he died.

My cousin got tested as well and she too was HIV-positive. Eight years ago, my cousin passed. We're not sure if she died from an overdose or something else. She was found in a pool of blood.

My Sister Story "Once was More than Enough"

Revelation

When she revealed that news, we were all scared. At the time, we really didn't know nothing about AIDS. We thought it was only something that homosexual men got. We did everything in our power to protect the kids from coming into contact with Sonya so she wouldn't spread the virus. She was adamant that they didn't eat or drink after her and she resigned from her job because she didn't want to infect the other kids.

As we became more and more educated about AIDS we discovered that just working around people didn't pass the virus (There are several ways to contract AIDS, unprotected sex, sharing a needle for drugs or steroids and blood transfusion and Mother to Baby during pregnancy, birth, or breastfeeding.)

As for myself I was extremely angry and mad that she lied about sleeping with Bobby. And the truth still dawns on me that she lost the apartment anyway, so she did it for nothing. She lived with her secret as long as she could before the debilitating disease began to have a toll on her physically and economically.

The emotional toll on her individual illness was even more frightening. Bills began to pile up unpaid because she was not able to work. Sonya went through an extremely difficult time in realizing that she was dying and there was nothing she could do about it.

My Sister Story "Once was More than Enough"

Life after Learning

And that's where the story begins. *My Sister's Story*. Once diagnosed with HIV everything changes and becomes different and new. Sonya turned into a cautious and careful person. She educated herself about the disease and learned as much as she could so that she would be able to take care of herself and made sure that she did not in fact cause and/or transmit the disease to anyone else.

When she found out that the virus could be translated via, sexual encounter, blood transfusion and sharing needles from drug uses, initially she thought it could only transmitted by sexual contact. She was still concerned that she could somehow touch a person and they too would get this debilitating virus. Once she quit working around kids she educated herself and realized that she couldn't pass the virus just by direct contact. She went back to work part time later after the diagnosis. During that time, she was dating a new guy. I'm not sure if he knew about her being HIV positive. He never discussed it with us.

The most important thing a person can do once they find out that they are indeed infected with this virus is to address this illness and at the same time share your diagnosis with your partner. Several cycles will pass through every person affected, first anger, then despondency and finally depression. Sonya became mad at the world and wondered why God chose her. She reasoned and rationalized that God was mad at her for backsliding. She felt God was punishing her for not trusting in him to meet her need.

It was funny, when you're confronted with something that you can't handle, the rationalizations, and the reasons that you create for being in that position in the first place. Faith, logic and reason goes out the window and you come up with idiotic answers to deal with the experiences that you're having mentally.

This challenge creates a mindset. This sets the stage on the way you look at things and the way you approach things.

My Sister Story "Once was More than Enough"

Mindset

One day the Lord placed upon my heart to turn my house into Sonya's house. A House of Refuge for women going through and dealing with AIDS and HIV. I turned over and questioned if the Lord was really speaking to me. After all I just finished raising my two children and was finally in a position where I could enjoy life myself. The urging in my spirit became so great that finally I relented and decided to turn my home into Sonya's House.

The days since that decision I've seen a lot of changes and challenges. My church Disciple Central Community Church, where Dr.

Marcus D. King is the senior pastor, was very supportive in the development of my nonprofit organization. Once the nonprofit status was granted I begin the process of turning my home into a place known as **Sonya's House Inc**.

Over the last year-and-a-half I have seen people from many walks of life make donations in cash, goods, services, and just time spent helping to develop this into a real dream come true. We've been able to build a Center that spreads education about AIDS and HIV as well as giving comfort and care to women going through the many stages of this disease.

I am often awed by how people are unselfish and so very caring and helping to someone that they don't even know or may never see. Every month supplies come in and the fundraising events are able to keep the doors open and meet the needs of the residents to come through.

The mindset of a community is changed when confronted with something so debilitating as AIDS or HIV. The human capital, as well as the monetary cost that are involved in treating and offering comfort to these young ladies can be monumental. I realize that many of these ladies are ostracized and polarized by their families and communities. They're often looked upon as being responsible for their own condition and therefore not qualified to receive the help and care that they so desperately need.

It has been my honor to be a catalyst for change in that Community. As I look at the pantry and the shelves that are stocked with everything necessary to make comfort and Kara possibility my spirit is lifted. To have a comfortable decent facility to provide these Services has been my dream since we lost someone so dear to us. The Legacy that I'm trying to provide in her name is that the care, and comfort that these ladies desire and deserve will be evident.

This Book is a combination of all of that and was designed to serve as a continual fundraising tool to be able to help not only the ladies of Sonya's house but also AIDS victims from around the world. My goal is to not only bring awareness to the disease but also to develop resources to help the victims not have such a low quality of life as they're living with this tragedy.

It's easy to sit back and point fingers at the decisions and choices made by people affected by AIDS. Initially it was thought that sexual transmission was the only way to contact this disease. Therefore it was easy to point fingers and blame. Now that we realize that other avenues such as blood transfusions and needle use can also spread this disease it becomes more of a moral equivalent to look at it and less than horrible turn.

We live in an age that is judgmental and critical about many things. My sister made a bad choice, others are making even worse choices every day. To exist in an environment where irresponsible sexual activity is commonplace, where drug use and other risky behavior is normal, makes those of us who never have had to experience that type of reality point fingers and pass judgment.

I never passed judgement on my sister, I was never ashamed of who she was or what she did. Of course I wish she never made that regrettable decision to sleep with Bobby, but more importantly I just wanted her to live. I wanted to have my sister close and be able to share all of the things that we shared together in our life.

As I look back I realized that except for the grace of God I could have been in her same situation that is one of the many reasons why I chose to give up my own home to turn it into a house in her memory. A house and a home that would be able to meet and exceed the needs that these women were facing similar situations find themselves confronted with.

The mindset of an individual living with AIDS or HIV is one of condemnation, torture, and disappointment. The depression that fills many of their days is born out because they realize that they made bad decisions. Those of us that are looking at their life to judge or condemn them are doing them and ourselves no favor.

One of the marks of a decent and moral person is that they see the least of us and seek to offer help and comfort. The Bible tells us that when we do it to the least of them we're doing it unto Christ. My intention in starting Sonya's House was to be able to do it to the least of them. The look in their eyes, the heartfelt appreciation for the services that we provide is thanks and reward enough.

To know that there's someone there to hold their hand and to offer them solace, comfort, care and encouragement during the worst time of their life is something that cannot be measured in money or reward.

Something larger than we as a family, something that speaks of the ideal of what Humanity is all about. It makes me feel good to know others have supported my vision. A tragedy like AIDs will confront and awaken either the best or the worst in us.

I lost my friend, and my sister. To lose the memories of what we spent and shared together would have been even more tragic. Thank you for taking time out of your life to read the story of my sister but also to contribute to making sure that all of our sisters across this land have an opportunity to live out what could become a nightmare, in a place of peace and solitude thank you.

My Sister Story "Once was More than Enough"

Prevention

I am not the moral police, it is not my job to tell you how to live your life. (Lord knows I have enough trouble trying to live mine right.) I do want to offer some simple tips on how to live an HIV/AIDS free life. It's very simple

1. Get tested early and often. You may be living a safe clean life but those that you interact with may not be

2. Always practice safe protected sexual activity. (Abstinence is best, but if you are active, be safe)

3. Do not share needles. (Drug abuse of any kind is not safe, but sharing needles puts you at far greater risk

4. Whereas infection from blood transfusions is not your fault, you still need to be proactive and get tested often to make sure if you inadvertently get infected, you can get treatment early enough to control or eradicate it

HIV infection happens in three stages. Without treatment, it will get worse over time and will eventually overwhelm your immune system.

First Stage: Acute HIV Infection

Most people don't know right away when they've been infected with HIV, but a short time later, they may have symptoms. This is when your body's immune system puts up a fight, typically within 2 to 6 weeks after you've gotten the virus. It's called acute retroviral syndrome or primary HIV infection.

The symptoms are similar to those of other viral illnesses, and they're often compared to the flu. They typically last a week or two and then completely go away. They include:

- <u>Headache</u>
- <u>Diarrhea</u>
- <u>Nausea and vomiting</u>
- <u>Fatigue</u>
- Aching muscles
- <u>Sore throat</u>
- <u>Swollen lymph nodes</u>
- A red <u>rash</u> that doesn't <u>itch</u>, usually on your torso
- <u>Fever</u>

Doctors can now prevent HIV from taking hold in your body if they act quickly. People who may have been infected; for example, had unprotected sex with someone who is HIV-positive, can take anti-HIV drugs to protect themselves.

This is called **PEP.** But you must start the process within 72 hours of when you were exposed, and the medicines can have unpleasant side effects.

My Sister Story "Once was More than Enough"

Second Stage: Chronic HIV Infection

After your immune system loses the battle with HIV, the flu like symptoms will go away. Doctors may call this the asymptomatic or clinical latent period. Most people don't have symptoms you can see or feel. You may not realize you're infected and can pass HIV on to others. This stage can last 10 years or more.

During this time, untreated HIV will be killing CD4 T-cells and destroying your immune system. Your doctor can check how many you have with blood tests **(normal counts are between 450 and 1,400 cells per microliter).** As the number drops, you become vulnerable to other infections.

Fortunately, a combination, or "cocktail," of medications can help fight HIV, rebuild your immune system, and prevent spreading the virus. If you're taking medications and have healthy habits, your HIV infection may not progress further.

Third Stage: AIDS

AIDS is the advanced stage of HIV infection. This is usually when your CD4 T-cell number drops below 200. You can also be diagnosed with AIDS if you have an "AIDS defining illness "such as Kaposi's Sarcoma or Pneumocystis Pneumonia

If you didn't know you were infected with HIV earlier, you may realize it after you have some of these symptoms:

- Being <u>tired</u> all of the time
- <u>Swollen lymph nodes</u> in your neck or groin
- Fever that lasts for more than 10 days
- <u>Night sweats</u>
- Unexplained weight loss
- Purplish spots on your <u>skin</u> that don't go away
- Shortness of breath
- Severe, long-lasting diarrhea
- <u>Yeast infections</u> in your <u>mouth</u>, throat, or <u>vagina</u>
- <u>Bruises</u> or bleeding you can't explain

People with AIDS who don't take medication only survive about 3 years, even less if they get a dangerous infection. But with the right treatment and a healthy lifestyle, you can live a long time.

(Source Web MD)

Chronic HIV

After acute infection, HIV is considered "chronic." This means that the disease is ongoing. Symptoms of chronic HIV can vary. There can be long periods of chronic infection when the virus is present but symptoms are minimal. In more advanced stages of chronic infection, symptoms can be much more severe than in ARS. People with advanced, chronic HIV can experience episodes of:

- coughing or breathing difficulties
- weight loss
- diarrhea
- fatigue
- high fever

My Sister Story "Once was More than Enough"

AIDS Is the Final Stage

Controlling HIV with medications is crucial to both quality of life and to help prevent a rapid progression of the disease.

Acquired Immune Deficiency syndrome (AIDS) develops when HIV has significantly weakened the immune system. According to the **CDC, Centers for Disease Control** this occurs when CD4 levels decrease below 200 cells per cubic milliliter of blood (mm3). A normal range is considered 500 to 1,600 cells/mm3. AIDS can be diagnosed with a blood test to measure CD4, but sometimes it's also determined simply by your overall health, particularly the presence of certain infections that are rare in persons with a normal immune system. Symptoms of AIDS include:

- persistent high fevers of over 100 degrees Fahrenheit
- severe chills and night sweats
- white spots in the mouth
- genital or anal sores
- severe fatigue
- rashes that can be brown, red, purple, or pink in color
- regular coughing and breathing problems
- significant weight loss
- persistent headaches
- memory problems
- pneumonia

Without treating HIV, the <u>Mayo Clinic</u> says that most patients develop AIDS within 10 years. At this point, your body is susceptible to a wide range of infections and cannot effectively fight them off. Medical intervention is necessary to treat infections or else death can occur. Without treatments, the <u>CDC</u> estimates the average survival rate to be three years once AIDS is diagnosed. Depending on the severity of infection, prognosis may be significantly shorter.

The key to surviving HIV and AIDS is to continue seeing your doctor for regular treatments. You should also schedule a visit as you experience new or worsening symptoms.

About the Author

BIOGRAPHY
NICKY HAWKINS

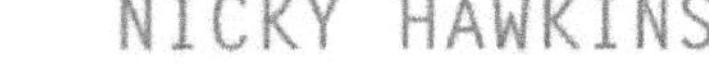

#StyledByNickyHawkins is the brain child of the beautiful and fashionably fierce, Nicky Hawkins.

Nicky Hawkins was born and raised in Dallas, Texas. She is a hard working soon to be, fashion mogul and the proud mother of two. Her love for fashion started at a very young age. Her sister Sonya was a "fashionista". "She would always tell me to never go outside without my hair done and clothes looking well put together." And to this day, even after her sisters passing, she still hears those words in her head loud and clear. "I remember when I was younger, I would sneak my sisters clothes and shoes out her room and wear them to school! The shoe's were too big and all but, I still wore them and I still looked good!" Nicky's passion for fashion has sentimental value to her and she loves the idea of sharing a little piece of her sister with the world.

#StyledByNickyHawkins is a consulting company whose motto is, "Fashion is the imagination, the clothes are the key to it!" Nicky believes that fashion is indeed a way of life and that it is one of the greatest forms of self expression. "Your appearance is the first representation of you. So, no matter what, do your best to look good! And don't be fooled, looking good doesn't take a million dollars. All it takes is an eye for fashion. And if you don't have that eye, well, thats what you have me for!"

In 2010 Nicky Hawkins opened up Starz Boutique in Duncanville, Texas. Starz Boutique was a women's only boutique and salon. Nicky's passion for making women feel beautiful inside and out set her on a mission to do just that. "I started personal shopping for my clients that never had time to shop for themselves." Unfortunately Nicky had to close her boutique. The closing of the boutique was earth shattering news for herself as well as her clients. Luckily that set back did not stop her, Nicky came back bigger and better. Nicky took that opportunity to create lasting relationships with stores and vendors. With those connections she is able to ensure that her clients always look and feel their best at all times.

Nicky specializes in image consulting, personal shopping, wardrobe styling, closet audits, personal styling, fashion workshops, closet organization, out of town packing, and bridal assistance. When it comes to looking amazing she is definitely the go to person. Not only is she good and what she does, she loves it!